CONT

INTRODUCTION

If you want to experience less back or neck pain you have to take back control over it by following the instructions through this book intensely and consistently.

As you know, it's not easy to determine the most effective treatment for your back pain. Differing opinions and information surrounding back pain create confusion and doubt in our minds. This overdose of information has led to uncertainty about the best path to healing neck and back pain.

This book will show you how to feel less pain, but it won't happen overnight or without effort from you. Through my experience over many years as a physiotherapist, I have seen many different causes for my patients' back pain, and more than anything, I want you to find what you have been missing.

Think of this book as your road map to a life without pain. A life where everyday stuff is easier to do, like putting your socks on in the morning, picking up something from the floor or putting the kids in the car. It's the life that you have wanted to live for a long time.

The goal of this book is to get you started in the right direction. The philosophy behind it is based on the premise that your pain is affected by both your mind and your body. Reading this book will give you a solid foundation of knowledge and proven back-relieving exercises. By committing to this simple exercise programme, you'll establish healthy new habits that you can build on throughout your life.

INTRODUCTION

Who is this book for?

This book was written for everyone who is struggling with neck and back pain in their everyday life, and for people who have tried all sorts of treatments or medications and yet have seen no lasting results, or worse yet, have experienced a steady increase in their pain and decline in their everyday function.

What you'll learn from this book

After reading this book, you will have learned:

How to break the fear and anxiety cycle that keeps you in a vulnerable and painful state;

- A new understanding of how our spine and body works
- How to increase your confidence levels through exercise
- How to identify muscular tightness and imbalances
- Ways to improve your posture
- Ways to use stretching to ease the build-up of tense muscles
- How to gradually strengthen your back muscles as you continue to gain confidence and regain your full range of activity

This book is broken down into two basic parts;

- **Part 1** will dispel the myths and confusion about back pain and help you to finally understand the real causes of everyday neck and back pain.

- **Part 2** will teach you the safe and effective neck and back exercises that increase flexibility and strength to the spine and surrounding muscles.

The best course of action is to read Part 1, not once but a few times to fully comprehend how the information relates to you and your pain. This will increase your understanding and confidence in your back before you start Part 2 and the exercise programme. Both parts of the book contain essential information for achieving long-lasting pain relief.

Your pain will lessen when you increase your knowledge and understanding of your pain and take the time and effort to work through the exercises. This is not an instant fix to your pain, but a long, steady road to recovery.

A quick browse through Part 1 and a couple of days of doing a few exercises isn't going to make much of a dent in the many processes that have caused your pain. I say this not to scare you, but to make sure you understand that it will take time and effort to achieve results.

If you are reading this book, you are probably in a negative mindset that includes:

- Being scared and confused about what is causing your pain
- Not knowing how to help ease your pain
- Being confused about which exercises are best to ease and prevent pain
- Lacking motivation and the 'get up and go' to do something about your pain

How do you move away from this negative mindset to embrace a strong, healthy outlook? See the next page for strategies to help you get and stay motivated.

INTRODUCTION

Strategy 1: Set Goals

Your motivation should be directly linked to a plan of action. If you're not clear on where you are going and how you are going to get there, you are setting yourself up for a fall.

Your goals should be specific and measurable. For example, let's say that in a specified period of time you want to be able to walk for 30 minutes, be able to play football with the kids or even to be able to put your socks on in the morning.

For best results establish short, intermediate and long-term goals. Here are some examples of each:

Short-Term Goal: "I want to establish a back exercise regime, slowly increasing my repetitions to ten over the next month."

Intermediate Goal: "In three months, I want to be able to walk the kids to school and vacuum the house."

Long-Term Goal: "In six months' time, I want to be able to go back to my old class in the gym."

To achieve these objectives, set yourself daily goals. You must take specific actions that are in line with your longer-range objectives. Each day, set yourself a plan:

- Know which exercises and how many repetitions you are going to do.
- Plan how many minutes of aerobic exercise you will do that day.
- Don't forget to congratulate yourself and be proud of your achievements when you complete your daily or weekly goals.
- Discipline yourself to keep a back exercise journal.

Remember you wouldn't be reading this if you didn't want to get back to the life you want!

Strategy 2: Remain Focused

At first, your body will want to resist the changes you are going to make. It is the body's natural urge to maintain the status quo by raising physical defences to unfamiliar physical exertion. For the first few days, your muscles and joints will feel tight and sore. Remember that the exercise programme is designed to progress at a slow, gradual pace.

Strategy 3: Form Partnerships

If you know someone who experiences similar pain and problems to yourself, such as a friend, work colleague of even your partner, encourage them to join you in reading this book, setting goals and going through the back exercise programme together. Having someone to share the experience with you can help keep you both on the right track.

Strategy 4: Accept Setbacks

During your path to recovery, you may have the odd bad day when you really ache. Accept this as part of the process, pace your activities that day and resume the programme as soon as possible. The longer you stick with the programme, the fewer setbacks you will experience.

Before you begin working towards your goals, you need to be in the right state of mind. In Part One of this book, we'll explore the powerful role your mind plays in helping you recover from the physical manifestations of back pain.

CHANGING PART 1
YOUR MIND

CHANGING YOUR MIND

Back pain has reached epidemic proportions in the western world. Today, an astonishing eight out of every 10 people are affected by this condition. Whether it affects the neck, shoulders, low back or upper buttock area, it can have a crippling effect on every aspect of a person's life. It can affect their ability to work and earn a living, enjoy recreational activities and participate fully in life. And it can affect their emotional and mental wellbeing, leaving them fearful, frustrated and hopeless.

Modern medicine: improved diagnostics, worsening outcomes

Why has the prevalence of back pain continued to rise, even as modern diagnostic and treatment options become more and more sophisticated and widely available? Magnetic resonance imaging (MRI), electromyogram (EMG) and myelograms allow doctors to see our muscles, nerves, bones and spinal canal and accurately pinpoint abnormalities that can cause pain. Every hidden element of our physical condition can be mapped and analysed, yet the majority of us continue to be plagued by pain and immobility. Why isn't modern medicine able to help?

The answer lies in the fact that modern medicine focuses exclusively on the physical dimensions of back pain. Elaborate diagnostic equipment is designed to lay bare the innermost workings of the human body and uncover structural abnormalities in the spine. The prescribed treatments are then based on addressing those abnormalities.

The entire diagnostic and treatment cycle deals only with the physical manifestations of the condition.

CHANGING YOUR MIND

In this conventional diagnostic/treatment cycle, the root causes of those physical problems remain unexamined and unresolved. It's no wonder that so many back pain patients experience unpredictable treatment outcomes! And it's no wonder that doctors and their patients have become so pessimistic about the possibility of long-term success in treating back pain.

Treating the hidden, emotional roots of back pain

The idea that a physical condition can also have an emotional component is difficult for some people to believe. But as our pain becomes ingrained in our mind and body, our perception of the pain changes along with our behaviour towards it. These changes in our minds and bodies create a chronic pain cycle. Emotional tension also has a proven ability to induce physiological change, including soft tissue damage that expresses itself as muscular tension and simple back strains. This soft tissue trauma is by far the most common cause of back pain.

In the same way that emotional stress can suppress our immune systems and affect our resilience to disease, it can have a destructive impact on our vulnerable soft tissue structures. This is why treatments based on physical assessment has failed time and time again to cure back pain permanently.

CHANGING YOUR MIND

Knowledge is the key to recovery

Successful and permanent treatment for back pain must be based on educating back pain sufferers. By teaching them to recognise and change these deep, ingrained perceptions and beliefs in their pain and the resulting emotional stress this produces, we can help them address and neutralise the real trigger for muscle tension and soft tissue damage. This holistic approach, which treats back pain as a physical, mental and emotional issue, offers a more effective and lasting treatment option. By training the pain sufferer to recognise and change their perceptions and beliefs, we are able to add a powerful psychological dimension to existing, physically based treatment options.

This book is designed to educate the reader about the emotional origins of back pain and provide a clear set of guidelines for healing back pain and managing emotional stress. As you read, you will learn to recognise how your own pain has a damaging emotional pattern. You'll also learn to use simple techniques to change them before they can affect your physical condition. You'll gradually be able to master these psychological stressors completely, and recognise your pain as harmless muscle tension that can be dissolved through knowledge, exercise and relaxation.

With the techniques you learn in this book, you are going to win your battle against back pain!

CHANGING YOUR MIND

You'll learn:

- Why the world of medicine offers little relief from back pain
- Why x-rays and MRI seldom correlate to patient symptoms
- Why only you have the power to control your recovery
- How to overcome fear and vulnerability
- How to learn to "trust" your back again
- How to actively plan your recovery and guard against recurrence
- Clear and easy to understand back exercises

Plus you'll get a step-by-step guide to controlling your emotions, retraining your pain response and neutralising your back pain.

So read on, keep an open mind and be prepared to learn something new about your health!

The limits of modern medicine, and the power of the individual

Medical professionals are trained to see back pain in terms of injury or damage to the spine. When they treat a back pain patient, they immediately start looking for explanations that fit a diagnosis. They use machines designed to show them every nook and cranny of your nervous system, bone structure and musculature so that they can pinpoint the exact location of the physical abnormality that's causing you to suffer.

Unfortunately, this limited diagnostic criteria completely ignores the most common reason for back pain. Even worse, it can be responsible for causing more anxiety and worry in the patients mind!

CHANGING YOUR MIND

The vicious cycle of diagnosis, fear and recurrence

Because of the medical community's over-reliance on these diagnostic investigations, we are told that our pain is based on a physical, structural vulnerability. That's why most of us are used to perceiving our backs as weak and easily damaged. When a medical professional examines your back and reinforces this self-perception by telling you that your back is, indeed, fragile and in need of support and treatment, you are likely to accept what they tell you without question.

Not only do you accept the diagnosis, you internalise it and begin to worry and grow fearful. You become anxious about hurting your back further. You become depressed about your poor health and concerned about your future. This accumulation of anxiety and stress, in turn, causes the arrangement of your muscles, nerves, tendons and ligaments to tighten and change. And it is these changes that cause your back pain to flare up and recur again and again.

You are now locked in a vicious cycle of diagnosis, fear about the diagnosis, and a recurrence caused by the psychological stress of those fearful emotions. By seeking a cure for your pain, you have in fact only generated more worry and anxiety in your condition. The real irony is that these emotional tensions are almost certainly what triggered your pain in the first place!

The doctors have your best interests at heart, but they are trained to focus exclusively on the physical origins of back pain. Because of this, they concentrate on the physical expressions and not the root cause of your condition, which is often mental, emotional and therefore invisible to their diagnostic machinery.

CHANGING YOUR MIND

Because a traditional medical diagnosis can evoke a fearful reaction that, in turn, prolongs and worsens your pain, it is very important for you to be able to recognise and address the emotional reasons for back pain.

Do structural abnormalities cause back pain?

Ask any doctor whether abnormalities in the structure of the back cause pain, and they will say yes. But when you ask why the incidence of back pain has increased rapidly over the past 30 years, they don't have an answer. The reality is that these physical abnormalities were prevalent long before MRIs and other diagnostic tools were invented. What has changed is the number of patients being diagnosed. More and more people are being scanned, x-rayed and told: "There's something wrong." As a result, more and more people are succumbing to anxiety about their condition, and that anxiety is creating a wave of Tension Related Pain (TRP).

Most of us have structural abnormalities in our backs. Everyone's back is different and develops in different ways as we grow and age. Everyone's back has been subjected to the stress of physical activity, trauma, health changes and other effects. But those structural abnormalities don't necessarily cause back pain. It's very important for back pain sufferers to understand that almost all spinal abnormalities are harmless.

TRP = Tension Related Pain

CHANGING YOUR MIND

Here are some examples of structural abnormalities:

Herniated discs: Our discs often wear out by the time we reach the age of 20. It's a perfectly normal (and harmless) part of the aging process, and an inevitable effect of gravity.

Low-back and shoulder pain: Recurring pain is most common in these areas. Revealingly, these areas are also the most likely to be the site of soft tissue (muscular) damage and tenderness cause by emotional tension.

Nerve damage: The sharp burning, tingling or numbness that accompanies nerve damage can be terrifying for the affected patient, but it is usually simply caused by pressure placed on the affected nerves by tense muscles.

In short, it's not the structural abnormalities that are causing pain, it's the stress of the prescribed diagnosis or of the unknown cause of your pain which manifests itself as TRP.

People often misdiagnose themselves, or accept a mistaken medical diagnosis that attributes their back pain to an injury that occurred long ago. The theory is that this old injury suddenly "flares up again" without reason. Alternatively, people believe that their pain is a result of a degenerative process, an abnormality or general weakness. Because the pain is physical, people automatically look for a cause that's physical. And of course, the prevalence of physical diagnostic equipment only feeds into that prejudice.

Let's take a look at this "vicious cycle" of misdiagnosis and worsening symptoms:

CHANGING YOUR MIND

Cycle of Pain, Misdiagnosis and Worsening Symptoms

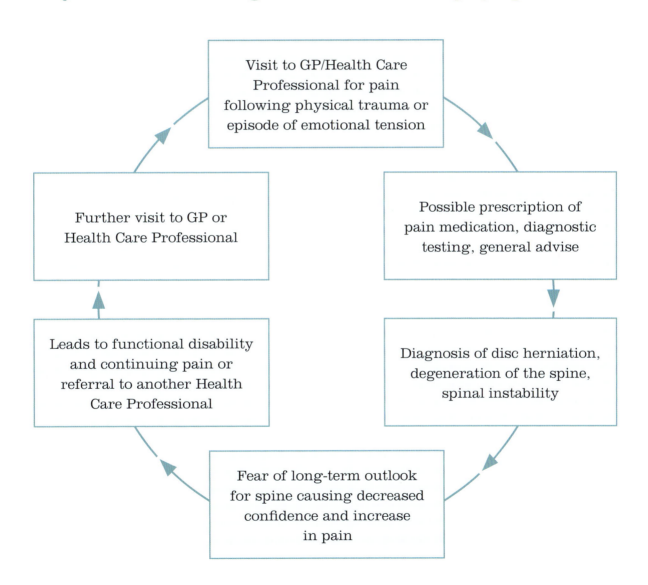

Visit to GP/Health Care Professional for pain following physical trauma or episode of emotional tension

Possible prescription of pain medication, diagnostic testing, general advise

Diagnosis of disc herniation, degeneration of the spine, spinal instability

Fear of long-term outlook for spine causing decreased confidence and increase in pain

Leads to functional disability and continuing pain or referral to another Health Care Professional

Further visit to GP or Health Care Professional

CHANGING YOUR MIND

Recognising Tension Related Pain

So, how can we recognise TRP and assess its impact on our back health and related pain levels? We can start by acknowledging sources of stress and tension in our lives.

Stress and tension can come from a number of areas of our life:

- Family conflicts and responsibilities
- Too much work and not enough support in the work environment
- Financial problems, debt and worries about the future
- Unresolved childhood issues of anger or low self-esteem
- Unrealistically high expectations for ourselves

If you can relate to any of these, scenarios, there is a good chance that you carry some level of harmful stress and tension in your body. This emotional stress then expresses itself in painful physical tension. This type of pain is most likely to show up in certain areas, including:

- Neck, top of shoulders and shoulder blades
- The lower back area
- Outer aspects of the buttocks

Tellingly, these are also areas that medical professionals identify as being most likely to be deprived of oxygen due to constricting muscular tightness, the kind of contraction that occurs with tension and emotional stress.

CHANGING YOUR MIND

Although these areas are very common sites of emotionally triggered pain, TRP can occur in other areas, and can also move around through the network of muscles, bones and nerves. Often, patients with TRP report pain that migrates to a new location as the old location starts to improve.

How do we stop the cycle of pain?

If conventional medical diagnosis and treatment is powerless to cure back pain, what methods can we use to stop the cycle of pain?

The first step in treating your pain effectively is to accept the psychological and emotional elements of your condition. Until you are willing to accept the role TRP plays in your back pain, you will never be able to reach the level of healing. You'll continue to be caught up in the vicious cycle of conventional diagnosis, fear, stress, and greater pain. Once you are ready to acknowledge that your physical pain may have an emotional origin, you will be able to open yourself up to a conscious program that involves training yourself to recognise and neutralise those damaging emotions. You'll be able to:

- Stop worrying about your pain
- Recognise your pre-programmed "pain patterns"
- Acknowledge and deal with your emotions
- Resist the urge to fall back on "physical" diagnoses

Let's take a closer look at each of these important steps.

CHANGING YOUR MIND

Stop worrying about your pain

After being incapacitated by back pain, it's hard not to worry when you feel a twinge. Even people who have never experienced back pain before are likely to react with fear after being told that back pain is caused by serious health issues. Most people react to the onset of back pain by imagining the worst that can happen—a degenerative condition, reduced mobility, missed work and weeks or months of pain.

However, it's important to resist the urge to wallow in fear and anxiety. The best thing you can do for your health is to overcome your apprehension, keep moving, and return to your normal activities.

Recognise your pre-programmed "pain patterns"

Did you know that you actively programme or condition your body to experience pain? By simply anticipating that a particular activity or situation will cause pain, you set up a pain pathway in your brain. For instance, you may assume that the act of getting in the car and driving is likely to cause a back flare-up—and sure enough, the next time you get into your car, you feel a twinge. Or perhaps you associate bending forwards or lifting things with back pain. You may have sustained a back injury whilst engaged in a particular activity, such as playing a sport. It's likely that whenever you play that sport in future, you hold anxiety about the possibility of a re-occurrence of back pain. These associations between a particular activity and the likelihood of pain are called "pain patterns," and they can actually cause you to bring on back pain through anxiety and stress.

Acknowledge and deal with your emotions

To deal with the impact of emotions on your physical health, you need to be

CHANGING YOUR MIND

honest about those emotions. If you are a worrier or a "type A" personality, overly responsible at home or at work, compulsive and a perfectionist, you need to acknowledge those traits in yourself. People most likely to suffer from TRP are often competitive, ambitious, goal-oriented and deeply driven to succeed. They put an intense pressure on themselves, which can lead to stress and anxiety.

Gaining an awareness of your psychological type and your tendency to internalise stress is critical in managing those pressures and controlling their effect on your back health. Think about how you deal with feelings of anger and anxiety. Sometimes, you may not even be aware that you hold those emotional tensions in your body, because they exist at the subconscious level. But it is helpful to ask yourself, "How do I deal with my emotions?"

For instance, try to be honest about how you deal with your anger. Do you tend to address it directly and try to resolve the issue? Or do you repress it and then release it at inappropriate times? If you hold repressed anger, you might have incidences of road rage in your past, or have a tendency to "snap" over small irritations.

The same is true of sadness, frustration, disappointment and a host of other negative emotions. If we don't handle our feelings in healthy ways, they create pools of tension in the body, this tension expresses itself as muscular pain. This pain, in turn, serves to distract attention away from the emotional realm and towards the physical realm. In this way, people subconsciously avoid dealing with their feelings, and instead expend their energies on coping with a physical complaint. Unfortunately, this means that they are unlikely to resolve their physical pain, as the emotional tension will surface again and again until it is addressed.

CHANGING YOUR MIND

Resist the urge to fall back on "physical" diagnoses

As mentioned earlier in this book, people have been taught for years that physical pain must have a physical cause. The medical profession reinforces this belief with a heavy reliance on structural diagnoses, such as MRI, CT scans and x-rays, which invariably interpret perfectly normal, degenerative changes in our spine as abnormal and painful conditions. These diagnoses, in turn, create crippling fears and anxieties that make us treat our backs as fragile, delicate structures that are prone to damage and require endless instructions on how to sit, stand, bend, work and lift.

As a result of this powerful and widespread misconception, most people will reject a diagnosis of TRP if it is presented to them. They refuse to believe that their pain is not only from a physical cause, and they fear that a TRP diagnosis somehow reveals them as being emotionally "weak." Unfortunately, our culture finds physical problems more acceptable that emotional or psychological ones.

Moreover, conventional diagnoses that identify physical degeneration as the source of their pain are so convincing. X-rays and scans seem so impressive to the patient, and doctors are so revered in our culture that it seems impossible that the pain could be caused by anything else.

What this means is that it's all too easy to turn away from an acceptance that TRP could be behind your back pain. But it's important that you keep an open mind and fully explore the possibility.

As many as 50 years ago, the groundbreaking neurologist Sigmund Freud said that many physical ailments had their basis in emotional tensions. For decades, the medical community chose to ignore these findings and focus exclusively on

CHANGING YOUR MIND

physical diagnoses. Today, in the face of irrefutable evidence, medical science is finally starting to accept the central role our emotions play in our overall health. New research is emerging almost every day about the interrelation between our minds and bodies. Science is only just beginning to untangle the ways in which the two affect one another, but the fact remains that they do, and you can use this knowledge to make a positive change in your quality of life!

Let's take a closer look at the relationship between emotional stress and TRP.

See flow chart page 26

So how do we prevent the formation of TRP in our bodies? How do we address the emotional basis of our pain and neutralise it before it manifests itself in pain, spasms and incapacitation?

We need to commit to a treatment plan that allows us to understand TRP, accept its role in our health, find ways to banish its effects and then use a combination of psychological and physical techniques to resolve our pain, once and for all.

Let's take a more detailed look at the four stages involved in treating TRP.

CHANGING YOUR MIND

How Tension Related Pain is produced in the body

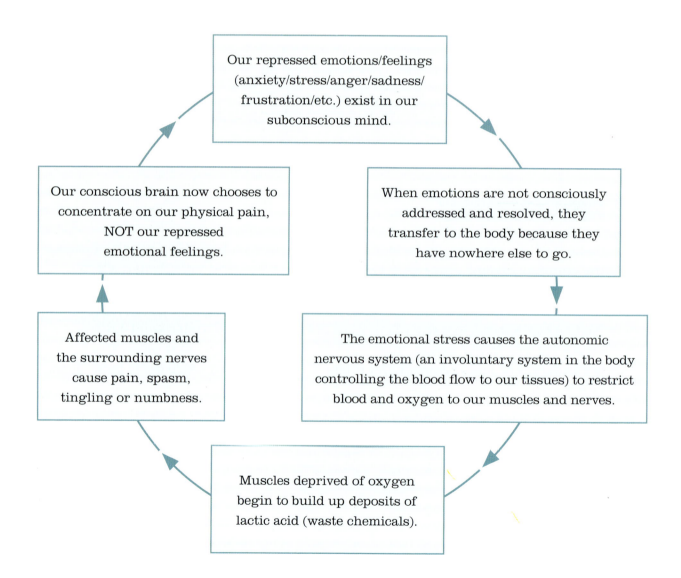

Our repressed emotions/feelings
(anxiety/stress/anger/sadness/
frustration/etc.) exist in our
subconscious mind.

Our conscious brain now chooses to
concentrate on our physical pain,
NOT our repressed
emotional feelings.

When emotions are not consciously
addressed and resolved, they
transfer to the body because they
have nowhere else to go.

Affected muscles and
the surrounding nerves
cause pain, spasm,
tingling or numbness.

The emotional stress causes the autonomic
nervous system (an involuntary system in the body
controlling the blood flow to our tissues) to restrict
blood and oxygen to our muscles and nerves.

Muscles deprived of oxygen
begin to build up deposits of
lactic acid (waste chemicals).

The Four Treatment Stages for TRP

Stage 1. Education and understanding

- Learn about Tension Related Pain (TRP)
- Learn how TRP affects the human body and causes pain

Stage 2. Acceptance of TRP and increased confidence of recovery

- Recognise the cycle of pain/diagnosis/fear/more pain
- Accept that your pain has an emotional root

Stage 3. Integration of new understanding into daily life

- Use exercise to stimulate blood flow and oxygen to areas of pain
- Start to return to previous activities with confidence
- Regain confidence and knowledge of how your body works and any imbalances in the muscles

Stage 4. Ongoing recovery and prevention

- Use awareness, acceptance and exercise integration together for the long-term resolution of your pain.

CHANGING YOUR MIND

Through these treatment stages, we approach your back pain in a holistic manner, with both mind and body engaged throughout. The mind/body approach includes:

1 **Knowledge therapy:** Educating yourself about TRP and fully accepting that your emotions can affect your physicality. Gaining awareness of your emotional patterns and re-programming your responses.

2 **Exercise therapy:** Building confidence, strengthening your spine and returning to full functionality and health.

Your treatment success will depend on your ability to maintain an open mind, a strong awareness of the ways in which mind and body interact, and a willingness to address and change your patterns of thought and behaviour. You must be ready to overturn decades of preconceived notions about physical health, and to see your pain as a symptom of a deeper, emotional state. Whenever you experience back pain, you will need to be able to see beyond the immediate pain and go further to examine the emotional state that triggered it.

Each time you feel a twinge of pain, you will need to train your attention away from the physical and towards an acceptance of the mental/emotional roots of your pain. Focus on ways in which everyday activity creates TRP within your body and how increased stress and anxiety in your everyday life increases TRP. It may take weeks or even months to be able to get beyond the immediacy of the pain and see deeper into the ultimate causes. Your mind is a very sophisticated machine, and it will not be easy to resist the tricks it can play on you. However, each time you make an effort to ignore the pain and focus on the real issues, you will be subtly shifting your brain patterns and making it easier, each time, to forge new pathways to the true source of your back pain.

CHANGING YOUR MIND

Tell your mind that you are in charge!

Each day, commit to making a conscious effort to see through the tricks your mind can play on you. Focus on your emotional state and the tension it creates in your body, rather than the specific area of pain. Remind yourself on a daily basis that you are actively engaged in a process of taking charge of your health and controlling the emotional states that create a false perception of pain.

Tell your body to get moving!

As you develop a new awareness of the root cause of your pain, you will begin to lose that familiar sense of fear about the condition of your back. You will stop feeling as through your spine is fragile and can be harmed by a single wrong move. You will start to feel stronger and more confident about moving naturally and freely. Instead of keeping yourself in a fear-based state of inactivity, you'll get up, move around and embrace a full and physically active life.

Once you truly accept that TRP is responsible for your back pain, your recovery will be gradual but steady. As you gain strength and vigour, you will begin to enjoy your exercise programme and see remarkable results.

By consciously fostering a hopeful attitude and a positive emotional outlook, you can learn to completely block pain and prevent it from recurring. This is a proven therapeutic process, and it will work for you if you give it the attention and commitment it deserves.

Can you imagine yourself healing your back through an integrated emotional/physical programme?

Then you're ready to move on to Part 2 of this book.

PART 2 THE ESSENTIAL EXERCISE GUIDE TO BACK & NECK PAIN

EXERCISE GUIDE

I could talk all day about back exercises. It's part of my daily job, and I love to help people on the road to recovery. I could show you hundreds of exercises that are easy to do and produce great results for my patients. But I know you don't have time or the patience to trawl through all these, so in this section, I have collected the most effective stretches and strengthening exercises for your neck, back, legs and arms. Each exercise targets a specific area quickly to help you gain confidence and mobility quickly. The programme also includes graduated back strengthening exercises to achieve excellent core and spine stability.

This is a complete, self-managed exercise guide designed to improve your back pain through integrated mind and body rehabilitation. You will learn to see your pain as harmless, encourage your body to shut pain off at the source, and return to a full and physically active life with confidence. Building on the knowledge you gained in the first half of the book, this programme will enable you to:

- Gain new understanding of how your spine and body works
- Increase your confidence in exercising
- Identify muscular tightness and imbalances
- Improve your posture
- Use stretching to ease the build-up of tense muscles
- Gradually strengthen your back muscles as you continue to gain confidence and regain your full range of activity

EXERCISE GUIDE

As a physiotherapist, I have assessed hundreds of patients with back pain, and every one of them was worried about the short- and long-term outcomes for their health. For many people, back pain is incredibly disabling, both in terms of the pain they experience and the restrictions the condition places on their mobility and independence. When someone has been in pain for months or even years, it often blots out their ability to think rationally about their condition. They feel panicked, fearful and pessimistic about the future of their health. It is at times like these that you need to keep in mind that pain does not equal harm.

The importance of pacing your return to exercise and fitness

If you have suffered from long term chronic back pain, you will need to start slowly when beginning the exercise programme, only performing a few repetitions and slowly increasing as you feel stronger. Think of it as a marathon, not a sprint, with a pain-free life waiting for you at the finish line. Slowly your confidence will improve and your muscles and joints will gain strength and mobility, allowing you to do the suggested number of repetitions. If you push your body too fast too soon, the ache in your muscles and joints will make you feel like giving up on the programme.

Just because you are in pain now, it doesn't mean that you are facing permanent disability or irreparable damage to your spine. As you discovered in the first part of this book, most causes of back pain is really a simple matter of emotional tension that affects the muscles and nerves, cutting off oxygen and creating painful constriction. Once you learn to control your emotional response to the pain, the tension will gradually release and leave you healthy, strong and whole. The programme requires an open mind, discipline, concentration and total commitment to influence a real and lasting change in your back health. Because the programme is based on a mental realignment as well as physical strengthening, positive envisioning techniques and mental exercises play a major role.

Not everyone sees results immediately. Depending on the type of back problems you have and your ability to overcome your fears and address the emotional issues underlying your pain, it may take weeks or even months before you are able to make a complete recovery. However, you will see results if you follow the programme faithfully and commit to adjusting your mindset

Let's begin!

MENTAL REHABILITATION EXERCISES

One of the biggest hurdles back pain sufferers face in overcoming their affliction is developing confidence in the power of their own minds. Just as they fear the physical weakness of their spine and back muscles, they fear that their own minds are just not strong enough to overcome the pain. I can promise you that your mind contains incredible power, and that you can harness that power to heal your own pain.

This is why a big part of the programme involves changing the way you think. By helping you build confidence in the power of your own mind, you will learn to see your back pain as a psychological, and physical issue. As such, it can be addressed by the power of the mind. By repeating key phrases that stimulate your mind to connect with the pain in positive ways, you will start the process of healing.

Each day, say the following things to yourself (silently or aloud):

- Structural abnormalities of the spine are the normal consequence of aging.
- My pain is a harmless condition due to mild oxygen deprivation.
- I can heal my pain through simple exercises, postural changes and renewed physical activity.
- I am not intimidated or afraid of my pain.
- By recognising and accepting TRP, I am well on my way to healing myself.
- I am in control of the pain, and I can choose to eliminate it by becoming more conscious of my pain patterns and emotional responses to stress.[1]

Over time, any doubts that are impeding your recover will begin to dissolve, and you will start to see a marked improvement in your physical condition. With every day that passes, you will find it easier and easier to see the effect your mental reconditioning has on your ability to manage and reduce pain.

BREATHING EXERCISES

If you find that you experience a setback, or just want a little extra support, it helps to discuss your healing journey with a family member or close friend. Breathing exercises are an incredibly important part of the programme, because they are a bridge between the mind and the body. Taking deep, even breaths is a purely physical act, yet it helps to put you in a more receptive, contemplative mental state. By becoming more aware of your breathing, you start to become more aware of the connection between you mind and your body. This helps you to become more confident in your mind's ability to affect your physical state.

Start by thinking about your breathing patterns. Do you tend to take shorter, shallower, more rapid breaths when you are tense or in pain? Shallow, rapid breathing can actually increase tension in your neck, shoulders and back, creating even more stress and pain. Concentrate on taking slower, deeper, more relaxed breaths. This will ease tension, reduce pain, and reinforce the relationship between a more relaxed state of mind and a healthier back.

See breating exercise page 36

References
1 Sarno, J. E., Healing Back Pain, The Mind-Body Connection. Warner Books, 1991.

BREATHING EXERCISE

Aim: To develop deeper, more relaxed, healthier breathing patterns

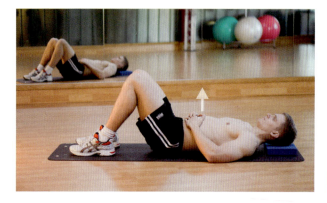
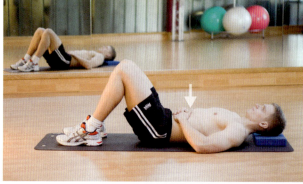

Starting Position:

Lie on your back on a mat or the carpet. Place a small, flat cushion or book under your head. Bend your knees and keep your feet straight and in line with your hips. Place your hands on your stomach. Keep your chest and ribcage relaxed and your chin gently tucked in.

Action:

1 Breathe in through the nose.
2 Feel your stomach filling with air and rising up.
3 Keep your head, neck and shoulders relaxed.
4 Ensure your shoulders are not rising as you breathe.
5 Breathe out through the mouth and feel your stomach flatten.

Repeat this breathing exercise throughout the day, in the car, office or at home, whenever you feel tension building.

Watch points

- Do not tense up through the neck and shoulders.
- Concentrate on using your diaphragm to breath.
- Imagine a small weight on your breastbone keeping it relaxed during the exercise.

MUSCLE IMBALANCE

A basic understanding of how our bodies work should be common knowledge for all of us, but it isn't!

If we have a nagging ache or pain, we should know how to stretch that area or muscle in order to aid the healing process. Unfortunately, most of us don't know how to use stretching exercises to address the onset of pain and keep ourselves limber.

Instead, most of us become less flexible as we get older. We start noticing that we can't touch our toes anymore, and one day we realise we even have difficulty putting socks on! Our muscles seem to tighten and tense up like boards.

You may be surprised to hear that age isn't the main culprit. A muscle's natural reaction is to contract. Muscles contract as a defense mechanism when they sense the onset of pain. In this way, our bodies develop habitual patterns of pain, which can also trigger a spasm attack.

Your muscles need balanced strength and flexibility to support your body height and weight and allow for normal movement. Unfortunately, for most of us, keeping all the muscles equally balanced is a tall order. We work some of our muscles too hard and allow other muscles to weaken, creating strength imbalances. We also over-stretch some of our muscles whilst leaving others to contract and become tense and tight. All of these tendencies lead to imbalanced posture over time.

Unfortunately, most people have no idea they're using their bodies in a way that creates imbalance. Let's look at some of the most common reasons for physical imbalance:

MUSCLE IMBALANCE

Lack of stretching

Most of us who do certain activities for long periods over and over again will lose flexibility if we don't adopt a regular stretching routine. This is because doing activities for extended periods of time cause some muscles to stay in a short, contracted state permanently, whilst others overstretch to compensate and become vulnerable to tearing and damage. Suddenly, we can no longer touch our toes or, in extreme cases, even our knees! To start your recovery, you need to address the muscle imbalances that causes conditions such as muscular tightness, disc herniation or spondylosis in the first place.

Sedentary lifestyle

If you sit for long periods, your muscles, tendons, and ligaments will adapt to this position. The result of this shortening causes tightness around joints, nerves or lengthened muscles that overstrain, creating imbalances in the body.

If you regularly spend long periods of time in front of a computer or television, behind the wheel, or at a desk writing or reading, the result will most likely be the weakening and stretching of your back muscles, rounded shoulders and a neck position that tilts or cranes forward. These effects lead to poor postures and muscle imbalances.

If you must lead a sedentary lifestyle, you need to sit with a square, straight-on posture, elbows by your sides, neck long and shoulder blades drawn into your spine. Make sure you get up at least once an hour to walk around, stretch, and loosen up. Get a glass of water, take a walk outside, perform a handful of stretches, or visit a colleague — anything to get your body moving.

MUSCLE IMBALANCE

Left- or right-handedness

Because so many of us are either left or right-handed, we tend to use one side of our bodies more than the other during our daily activities. This strengthens some muscles and leaves others underdeveloped and weak. To create a better balance throughout the body and better support for the spine and the back, start consciously using both sides of your body more evenly.

If you normally lift your child with your right arm, for example, or balance her on your right hip, try lifting her with your left arm and balancing her on your left hip. Bend your knees when lifting her and never carry her for too long on just one side. Get used to shifting and using more of your muscles. This will improve your overall body symmetry, strength and flexibility.

Most of us also tend to carry our possessions on one side, which can also cause problems. For instance, habitually wearing a shoulder bag on one shoulder causes your body to tilt and bend to compensate, straining your spine. It also forces the muscles on the carrying side to work harder than the ones on the other side. If you need to carry some sort of bag on your shoulder, be sure to frequently switch sides, so both shoulders are worked equally. Even better: use a rucksack that allows you to achieve balance between both sides of your body.

These chronic muscle imbalances are a major contributing factor to back pain. However, with the help of the exercises later in the book, you can self-assess the strength and flexibility of your muscle pairs in your hips, pelvis, spine, and throughout the body. The idea is to find out which muscles are strong and which are weak, which are tight and which are more flexible, and which may

MUSCLE IMBALANCE

be overworked or shortened. Since these various imbalances stress joints, other muscles, and ligaments, the goal of the therapy is to rebalance the muscles so that each muscle pair is as close to "normal" as possible. By evening out the muscle tension between the left and right sides of the body or between the front and back, the body supports the spine more evenly, automatically improving posture. This postural realignment allows the vertebrae to move back into position, taking pressure off irritated nerves and muscles and eliminating back pain.

As you can now see, your back pain is caused by a multitude of factors brought on over many years by physical and mental habits which have become the norm for your body. It will take time to break the cycle, but it can be done. Once you establish new, healthier daily physical and mental habits, your back pain will diminish and eventually disappear.

POSTURAL AWARENESS

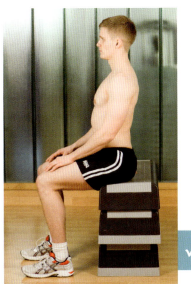

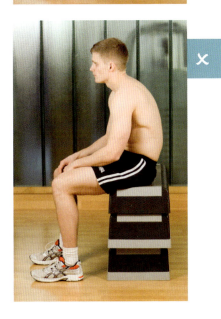

Postural awareness

Developing a keen awareness of your posture is one of the most effective ways you can strengthen your back and reduce muscle tension. Of course, the majority of us do not have perfect posture, and the misalignment of our spines can create areas where our emotional tensions can pool and create pain. When standing or sitting, it's important to be aware of any imbalances in the muscles or areas of stress. Once you develop this awareness, you can address these issues by adjusting your posture and practising the exercises to reinforce better posture. As your sitting and standing habits improve, you'll notice far less tension in your body and less strain on you soft tissues and spine.

Slumping: If you tend to slump in your chair, it generally means your low back is overstretched. As a result, your muscles and joints compensate, causing shortening to the soft tissues and imbalances throughout the spine.

POSTURAL AWARENESS

Let's look at this cycle in more depth.

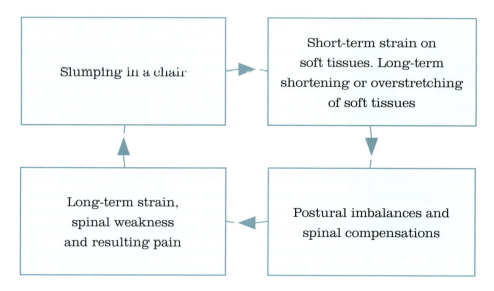

"Uptight" sitting postures

When we remain seated for long periods of time (for instance, seated at the computer or driving long distances), it can cause our muscles to contract and tighten, resulting in pain. Regular changes of position and gentle stretching, ideally every hour, will benefit our muscles and joints.

Uneven sitting postures

If you sit consistently with your legs crossed to a particular side, it can cause your lower back to curve sideways, putting strain on your soft tissues. Try switching sides each time you cross your legs to create more balance in your sitting posture.

POSTURAL AWARENESS

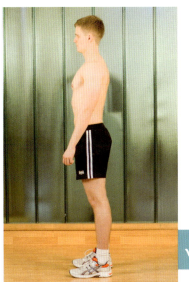

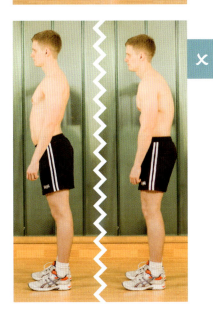

Standing posture

To determine whether your standing posture needs to be adjusted, stand in front of a full-length mirror. Stand sideways, and place your hands on your hip bones. Now, imagine your pelvis were a bowl of water, and feel the position of your hip bones. Are you tipping the "bowl" forwards or backwards, or are you holding it level? For ideal posture, you want to focus on keeping the imaginary bowl of water level. Focus on making slight postural adjustments until you achieve this effect. Now take a mental snapshot of how this looks, and remember how it feels to hold the posture.

Next, look at the way you hold your head and neck. You want to make sure your chin is tucked in slightly towards your chest, so that your neck is lengthened slightly. If your chin or head juts forward, gently pull yourself into alignment.

And finally, develop an awareness of whether you tend to favour one leg or another when you stand. If there is an imbalance in the way you distribute weight on your legs, make sure you change your weight-bearing leg regularly.

POSTURAL STRENGTHENING

Postural strengthening

Now that you have a greater awareness of your postural issues, you can begin to address those issues by strengthening your areas of weakness. Improving your posture through strengthening exercises is key to eliminating soft tissue imbalance and resulting pain. As part of your rehabilitation programme, commit to achieving these postural corrections throughout the day. If you can find healthier ways to stand and sit, it can radically change your back pain. After all, most people spend more hours in the day standing and sitting than they do in more active pursuits. Improving these two postural modes form an essential part of your overall back health.

"Protruding" posture exercises: If your abdomen and buttocks tend to protrude when you stand, it increases the arch in your lower back, creating imbalances in the muscles. To improve your posture, practice the Pelvic Tilt exercise on page 44 which can be done anywhere, at any time: using your abdominal muscles, gently tilt your pelvis backward and tuck in your tailbone. Repeat as many times as you like. This simple exercise helps realign a protruding posture and allows the back to relax.

Other helpful exercises for a protruding posture include:

POSTURAL STRENGTHENING

"Slumped" posture exercises: If you tend to slump forward when you stand, with your pelvis tilted backwards and your tailbone tucked under, you have a "slumped' posture. This posture can cause your shoulders to collapse inward, creating tension and pain. To improve your posture, try imagining that there is a string attached to the crown of your head, and that the string is being pulled upwards tautly. Allow the string to slowly pull you taller and straighter. Tuck in your chin, draw your shoulder blades down into your back, lift your chest and allow your neck to lengthen.

Other helpful exercises for a slumped posture include:

BACK PAIN TREATMENTS

This selection of treatments can help you manage pain whilst you focus on strengthening mental control over your pain and your exercise programme. Although the ultimate aim of the programme is to help you become pain-free so that you don't need these pain-management treatments, they are helpful to use as short-term, interim pain relief.

Cold treatment: Using ice packs on painful areas helps to reduce inflammation and calm the pain receptors. Apply ice for 10 minutes and repeat every two hours as needed.

(Precautions: wrap ice in thin towelling; if icing irritates symptoms, discontinue the treatment; if you have heart, circulatory or lung problems, decreased sensation or an open wound, consult a healthcare professional before commencing ice pack treatment.)

Heat treatment: Use heat packs, such as wheat bags, to help relax muscle spasms and tension. Apply heat pack for 20 minutes and repeat every two hours as needed. Even a hot shower over the painful area can help ease muscle tension.

(Precautions: use protective layers to protect the skin from excessive heat; follow the instructions on the heating product; if you have heart, circulatory or lung problems, decreased sensation or an open wound, consult a healthcare professional before commencing heat treatment.)

Soft tissue massage or self-massage: Gentle massage from a qualified massage therapist can help with pain relief. Self-massage can also be helpful. Try standing against the wall or lying on the floor and massage your muscles using tennis balls pressed gently between your tissues and the hard surface. A vibrating, hand-held massage device can also help relieve muscle tension and pain.

Bending and lifting advice: To use the right postural technique when bending and lifting, keep your feet shoulder width apart, bend your knees, and keep your chest up and your back straight. If you are lifting a heavy or awkward object, bend the knees and go into a half-kneeling position, keeping the weight drawn close to your chest. Never lift heavy objects repeatedly over a short period of time.

EXERCISE GUIDE

As you begin performing the exercises, aim to connect to your body mentally. When you stretch a muscle, concentrate on the sensation this creates within that muscle. Only move and stretch as far as is comfortable, and only take yourself into a position where you can breathe and relax into the movement.

Always listen to your body and learn the difference between the feeling you get when you stretch a tight sore muscle and the pain caused when you hurt yourself. If you feel a sharp stabbing pain when exercising, stop immediately.

These exercises will teach you discipline and control, and help you to connect your mind to your muscles. Ultimately, this will lead to you achieving the result that you want...less pain!

This exercise programme will take you from doing no back exercises to doing 20-30 minutes a day, enough to increase the flexibility and strength of your back and neck.

You may need to gradually increase the repetitions until you are able to follow the recommended amount. But if you persevere, you will gradually improve. Everyone is different, so adjust the exercises to fit your needs. If your neck and shoulder blades are the main problem, then concentrate on this area on a daily basis.

To help achieve the correct technique, each exercise is accompanied with a Watch Points section. To perform these exercises safely, make sure you check this section for each exercise.

The General Aerobic Exercise Programme will give you the confidence to get moving again and the motivation to return to those neglected pastimes you have been missing.

The most important consideration when learning these exercises is safety. If you have any health problems or concerns, you must consult a health care professional before you start the programme.

EXCERCISE PROGRAMME

TOP TIPS

- Follow the instructions for each exercise closely. You must learn the proper technique to achieve the best results.

- Keep an open mind. As you learn each exercise, your body will surprise you. Some stretches will feel difficult, some easy and some tight only on one side of your body! Adjust and adapt as you progress through the programme.

- Keep challenging your body. If you feel able to increase the repetitions, sets or levels for each exercise, then go for it.

- You must exercise consistently. Build a daily routine and stick with the programme. No excuses!

- Mix it up! Vary the exercises considerably during each week. Focus sometimes on stretches, sometimes on strength, sometimes general fitness. This will help keep you interested and motivated.

- Remember to work on your mental resilience at the same time as your physical programme. You must believe that your pain will get better.

- To keep yourself motivated, reward yourself with a little present if you complete the exercises each day for a month.

- When exercising, focus on the movements. Do not allow yourself to become distracted by anything or anyone.

- Be patient. We all get frustrated at not progressing faster at one time or another. Give your body the chance over the long term to reach your goals.

- Be realistic. You may not achieve a 100% pain free life. But you will achieve substantially less pain during your daily activities if you stick to your exercise programme.

LOW BACK STRETCHING

The stretches in this section focus on your low back. Over time, they help you improve the range of motion in your back in order to make everyday tasks easier.

Benefits of low back stretching

✓ Reduced tension in your muscles and joints

✓ Improved posture

✓ Less discomfort in your lower back

✓ A more comfortable body to walk around in all day

The Routine

■ If you suffer from low back pain, start off by practising each exercise to uncover any muscular tightness to the spine.

■ Identify three to five exercises that you feel best stretch your problem areas.

■ Do this routine every day.

■ Follow each exercise instruction and gradually increase to the recommended amount.

■ Keep each motion slow and controlled.

■ Remember to maintain abdominal breathing throughout the exercises.

KNEE TO CHEST STRETCH

Aim: To improve flexibility of your low back

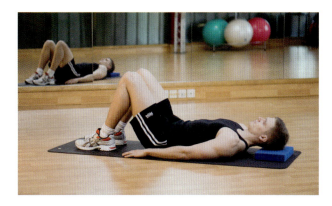

Starting Position:

Lie on your back on a mat or the carpet. Place a small flat cushion or book under your head. Bend your knees and keep your feet straight and in line with your hips. Keep your chest and ribcage relaxed and your chin gently tucked in.

Action:

Bend one knee up towards your chest and grasp with two hands behind your knee. Slowly increase this stretch as comfort allows. Hold for 20-30 seconds with controlled deep breaths.

Repeat three times, alternating legs.

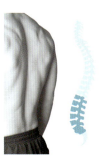

Watch points

- Do not tense up through the neck, chest or shoulders
- Only stretch as far as is comfortable

Variations: Grasp behind both knees and stretch into chest

CAT STRETCH

Aim: To mobilise and stretch the entire spine

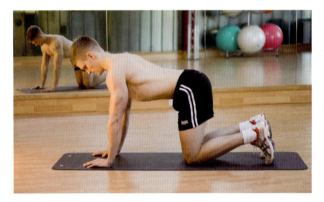 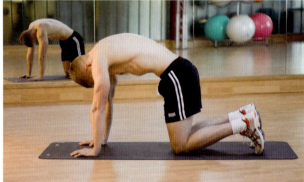

Starting Position:

Kneel on all fours, with your knees under hips and hands under shoulders. Make sure you keep a small inward curve in your low back. Keep your neck long, your shoulder blades down and your elbows unlocked.

Action:

Begin at the base of your spine, slowly tuck your tailbone under, work your way up the spine finishing with your chin on your chest and your spine in a C-shaped curve. Slowly uncurl the spine, leading from the tailbone vertebra by vertebra until you return to the starting position.

Repeat eight to 10 times.

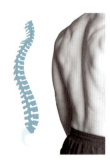

Watch points

- Concentrate on moving every vertebra segment by segment.
- Do not overarch downwards or lift up your head.

BOTTOM TO HEELS STRETCH

Aim: To stretch and mobilise the spine

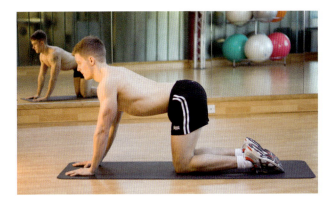

Starting Position:

Kneel on all fours, with your knees under hips and hands under shoulders. Make sure you keep a small inward curve in your low back. Keep your neck long, your shoulder blades down and your elbows unlocked.

Action:

Slowly take your bottom backwards keeping the natural curves in the spine. Only stretch as far as is comfortable. Hold the stretch for one deep breath and return to the starting position

Repeat eight to 10 times.

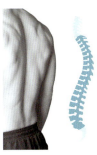

Watch points
- Avoid sitting back on your heels if you have a knee problem.
- Check your spinal alignment during the exercise with the help of a mirror.

KNEE ROLLS

Aim: To stretch and mobilise the spine

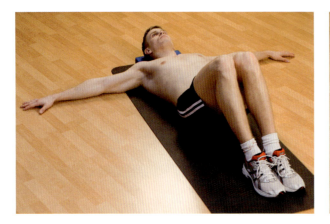 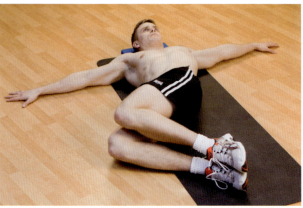

Starting Position:

Lie on your back on a mat or the carpet. Place a small flat cushion or book under your head. Keep your knees bent and together. Keep your chest and ribcage relaxed and your chin gently tucked in.

Action:

Roll your knees to one side, followed by your pelvis, keeping both shoulders on the floor. Hold the stretch for one deep breath and return to the starting position.

Repeat eight to 10 times, alternating sides.

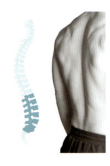

Watch points
- Do not move into pain only move as far as is comfortable.
- Place a pillow between your knees for comfort.

SCIATIC MOBILISING STRETCH

Aim: To mobilise the sciatic nerve and hamstrings

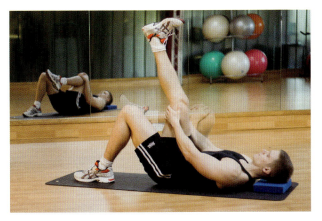

Starting Position:

Lie on your back on a mat or the carpet. Place a small flat cushion or book under your head. Bend your knees and keep your feet straight and in line with your hips. Keep your chest and ribcage relaxed and your chin gently tucked in.

Action:

Bend one knee upwards towards your chest and grasp with both hands behind the knee. Slowly straighten the knee whilst bringing your foot towards you. Hold for 20-30 seconds taking deep breathes. Bend the knee and return to the starting position.

Repeat alternating legs two or three times.

Warning!

If you suffer from **sciatica**, please seek advice from a medical professional before attempting this exercise.

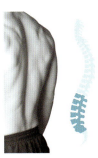

Watch points
- Do not press your low back down into the floor as you stretch.
- Only stretch as far as is comfortable, and stop immediately if you feel pain, numbness or tingling

BACK EXTENSIONS

Aim: To stretch and mobilise the spine backwards into extension

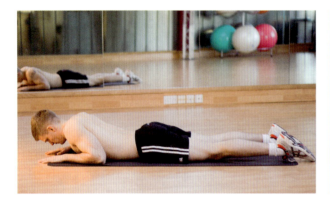
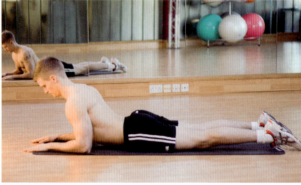

Starting Position:

Lie on your stomach, and prop yourself on your elbows extending your spine. Keep your neck long.

Action:

Gently keeping your neck long, extend your spine backwards, straightening your elbows if this feels comfortable. Hold for five to 10 seconds. Return to the starting position.

Repeat eight to 10 times.

Watch points
- Do not extend your neck backwards.
- Only extend as far as is comfortable.

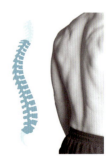

STANDING SIDE BENDS

Aim: To stretch the sides of the spine

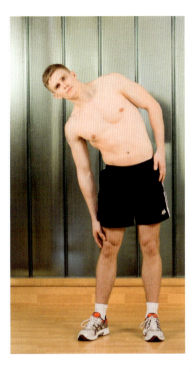
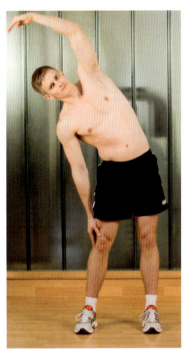

Starting Position:

Stand with your feet hip-distance apart and your spine in alignment. Place one hand on your hip and the other on the outside of the thigh. Keep equal weight through both feet during the exercise. Keep your neck long.

Action:

Slide the hand down the outside of the thigh, feeling the stretch on the opposite side. Return to the starting position.

Repeat, alternating sides eight to 10 times.

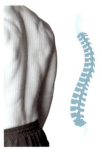

Watch points

- Only stretch as far as is comfortable.
- Take deep abdominal breaths throughout the exercise.
- Keep your weight equally distributed through both feet throughout
- Keep upright and do not bend forwards

Variations: Instead of keeping one hand on your hip, raise the arm above the head to increase the stretch.

SPINE ROTATIONS

Aim: To rotate the spine

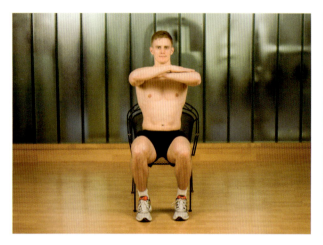 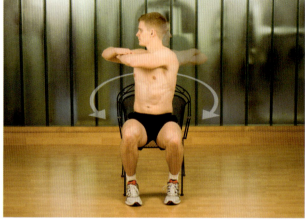

Starting Position:

Sit in a chair and fold your arms in front of you, in line with your chest. Keep your shoulders down and your neck long. Imagine a metal pole down your spine, which you rotate around.

Action:

Rotate to one side as far as is comfortable, whilst keeping your pelvis square. Slowly return to the starting position.

Repeat 8-10 times alternating sides

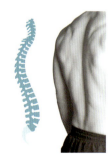

Watch points

- Keep equal weight through both buttocks.
- Concentrate on pivoting around the imaginary pole.
- Keep your shoulders down and neck long

LOW BACK
STRENGTHENING 1

In Level 1 of your strengthening programme, you will learn how to activate your deep abdominal muscles, low back muscles and buttocks. This will give you a solid foundation of muscles around your back in order to avoid further injury or re-occurrence.

Benefits of low back stretching

✓ Less discomfort in your lower back

✓ Everyday tasks will become easier

✓ More confidence in your back to take on new challenges

✓ Improved posture

The Routine

■ Start the Level 1 exercises and follow each exercise instruction and gradually increase to the recommended amount.

■ Keep each motion slow and controlled.

■ Remember to retain the abdominal breathing throughout the exercises.

■ Between exercises, try to rest for no longer than five seconds.

■ Even if you find Level 1 easy, make a point of practising these exercises every day for at least two weeks. It is important to lay a firm groundwork before progressing to Level 2.

■ If you need more time, stick with Level 1 beyond the first two weeks.

■ After two weeks, if you have achieved the recommended repetitions and sets, you can progress confidently to Level 2.

DEEP ABDOMINAL STRENGTHENING

Aim: To strengthen the deep supporting muscles surrounding the spine

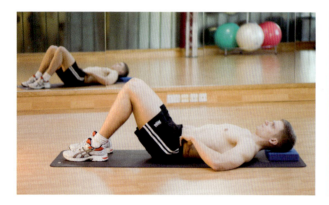
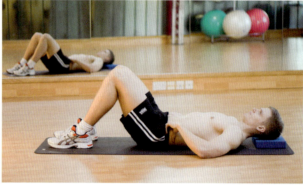

Starting Position:

Lie on your back on a mat or the carpet. Place a small, flat cushion or book under your head. Bend your knees and keep your feet straight and in line with your hips. Keep your chest and ribcage relaxed and your chin gently tucked in. Once you have mastered this technique, keep practising in differing positions throughout the day.

Action:

As you breathe out, draw up the muscles of the pelvic floor and lower abdominals, as though you were doing up an imaginary internal zipper! Hold this gentle muscle contraction whilst practising your abdominal breathing for five to 10 breaths.

Repeat five times

Watch points
- Remember, this is a slow, gentle tightening of the deep abdominal muscles. Do not pull these muscles in using more than 25 per cent of your maximum strength.
- Make sure you do not tense up through the neck, shoulders or legs.

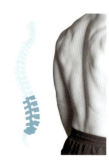

Aim: To stretch and strengthen the low back

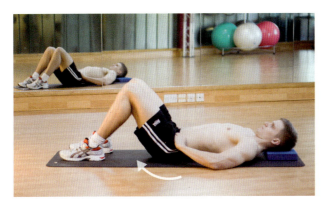 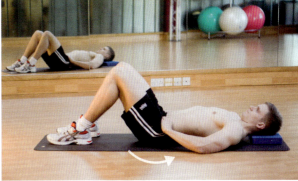

Starting Position:

Lie on your back on a mat or the carpet. Place a small, flat cushion or book under your head. Bend your knees and keep your feet straight and in line with your hips. Keep your chest and ribcage relaxed and your chin gently tucked in.

Action:

Gently tuck your tailbone under you whilst simultaneously contracting your stomach muscles. Feel your ribcage draw towards your pelvis and your low back gently press down into the mat. Now, return to the starting position and then slowly arch your back, feeling the low back muscles working.

Repeat eight to 10 times

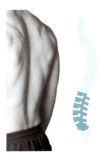

Watch points
- Only stretch as far as is comfortable.
- Take deep abdominal breaths throughout the exercise.
- Do not push down through you feet during the exercise.

Modifications: Place one hand on your stomach and the other under your low back and use this feedback to feel the correct muscles working.

LEG SLIDES

Aim: To strengthen the supporting muscles surrounding the spine

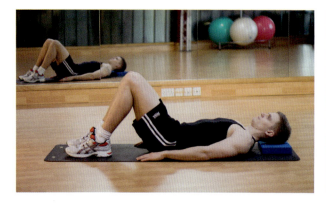
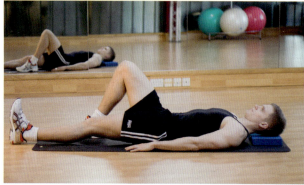

Starting Position:

Lie on your back on a mat or the carpet. Place a small, flat cushion or book under your head. Bend your knees and keep your feet straight and in line with your hips. Keep your chest and ribcage relaxed and your chin gently tucked in.

Action:

Slide one leg along the floor, keeping your back still and deep abdominals engaged. Return the leg to the bent position whilst carefully keeping your low back still.

Repeat eight to 10 times, alternating legs.

Watch points
- Keep your deep abdominals activated throughout
- Do not let your low back arch
- Do not tense up through the chest, shoulders or neck

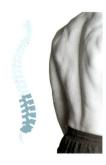

KNEE DROPS

Aim: To strengthen the supporting muscles surrounding the spine

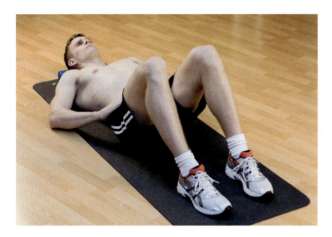
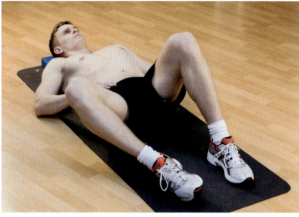

Starting Position:

Lie on your back on a mat or the carpet. Place a small, flat cushion or book under your head. Bend your knees and keep your feet straight and in line with your hips. Keep your chest and ribcage relaxed and your chin gently tucked in.

Action:

Allow one knee to drop slowly outwards whilst keeping your pelvis stationary. Draw the knee back in towards your body.

Repeat eight to 10 times, alternating legs.

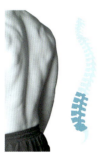

Watch points
- Keep your deep abdominals activated throughout
- Imagine a spirit level across your hipbones and keep this level at all times
- Do not tense up through the chest, shoulders or neck

LEG LIFTS

Aim: To strengthen the supporting muscles surrounding the spine

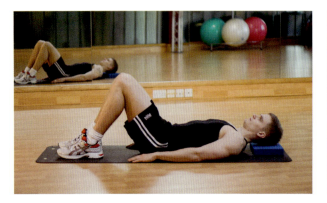
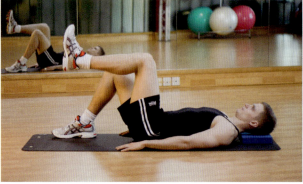

Starting Position:

Lie on your back on a mat or the carpet. Place a small, flat cushion or book under your head. Bend your knees and keep your feet straight and in line with your hips. Keep your chest and ribcage relaxed and your chin gently tucked in.

Action:

Slide one foot back and then lift this leg up until your lower leg is horizontal. Lower the leg to the starting position.

Repeat eight to 10 times, alternating legs.

Watch points
- Keep your deep abdominals activated throughout.
- Do not let your low back arch.
- Do not tense up through the chest, shoulders or neck.
- Make sure you do not tense up through the neck, shoulders or legs.

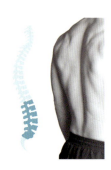

SWIMMING

Aim: To strengthen the low back and buttocks

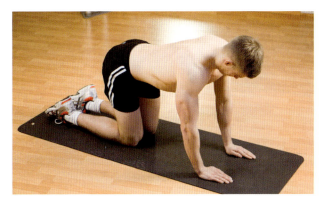

Starting Position:

Kneel on all fours, with knees under hips and hands under shoulders. Make sure you keep a small, inward curve in your low back. Keep your neck long, your shoulder blades down and your elbows unlocked.

Action:

Reach one arm forwards off the floor as far as control can be maintained through your pelvis and low back. Repeat with the other arm. Slide one foot along the floor away from the body. Continue to reach and raise the leg off the floor as far as control can be maintained. Repeat with the other leg.

Repeat alternating arms eight to 10 times and repeat with the legs

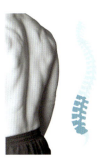

Watch points
- Keep you neck long and deep abdominals activated throughout.
- Keep the correct curvature throughout the spine during the exercise.
- Lengthen and raise the leg by activating the buttocks Imagine a glass of water on your back throughout the exercise

BRIDGING

Aim: To improve flexibility and stability of the spine

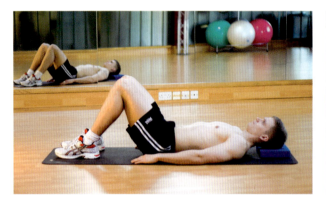
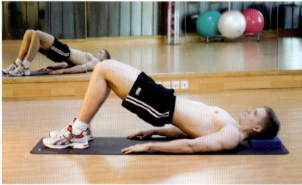

Starting Position:

Lie on your back on a mat or the carpet. Place a small, flat cushion or book under your head. Bend your knees and keep your feet straight and in line with your hips. Keep your chest and ribcage relaxed and your chin gently tucked in.

Action:

Activate your deep spinal muscles and gently roll your lower back into the mat. Scoop your tailbone upwards and continue to peel your spine off the mat, vertebra by vertebra, until you are resting on your shoulder blades. Achieve this by squeezing your buttocks during elevation. Lower one vertebra at a time onto the mat, beginning with the highest and finishing with your tailbone.

Repeat eight to 10 times

Watch points
- Keep your deep abdominals activated throughout.
- Keep your neck long and relaxed.
- Relax your ribcage and do not push your chest forwards.
- Work through the buttocks not through the hamstrings.

Variations: Gently squeeze a towel or cushion between your knees.

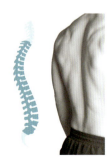

SIDE-LYING LEG RAISE

Aim: To strengthen the buttocks and low back

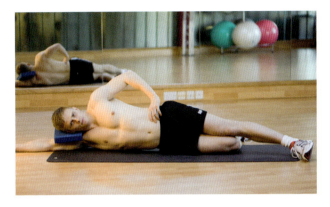
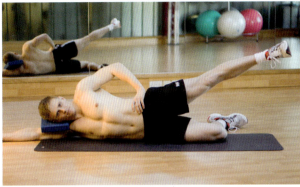

Starting Position:

Lie on your side with your bottom knee bent to 90 degrees and your top leg straight and in line with your spine. Keep your hips stacked on top of each other. Gently press with your fingers into the muscle of your upper buttock (in the area where the back pocket of your trousers would be) to keep your hip forward.

Action:

Raise the top leg towards the ceiling. Do not let your pelvis roll backwards. Slowly lower to the starting position.

Repeat eight to 10 times on one side, then change sides and repeat.

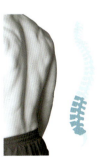

Watch points

- Keep your top hip forward throughout the exercise
- Raise your leg in line with your spine.
- Keep your deep abdominals activated throughout.
- Use a mirror to check your alignment during the exercise.

LOW BACK STRENGTHENING

Now that you have a solid foundation around your spine by achieving Level 1, you can challenge your back and build further strength and control with these advanced exercises.

Benefits of Low Back Strengthening Level 2

✓ Increased strength and endurance in your abdominals and low back

✓ Improved posture

✓ Confidence to return to your previous sport or activities

✓ Improved body awareness and muscle activation

The Routine

■ Start the Level 2 exercises, follow each exercise instruction and gradually increase to the recommended amount of repetitions.

■ Repeat Level 2 exercises every other day, in order to allow your muscles to fully recover from their workout.

■ Between exercises, try to rest for no longer than five seconds.

■ Keep each motion slow and controlled.

■ Remember to retain the abdominal breathing throughout the exercises.

BRIDGING

Aim: To improve flexibility and stability of the spine

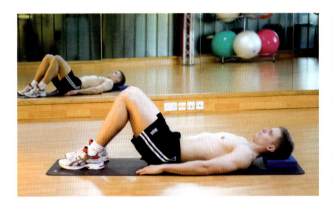
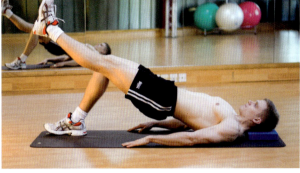

Starting Position:

Lie on your back on a mat or the carpet. Place a small, flat cushion or book under your head. Bend your knees and keep your feet straight and in line with your hips. Keep your chest and ribcage relaxed and your chin gently tucked in.

Action:

After raising the spine off the floor, straighten one leg and slowly lower it, just as you did for Bridging Level 1.

Repeat, alternating legs, eight to 10 times.

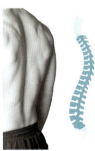

Watch points
- Keep your deep abdominals activated throughout
- Keep both sides of your pelvis level and do not allow one side to dip whilst straightening one knee

2 SWIMMING

Aim: To strengthen the low back and buttocks

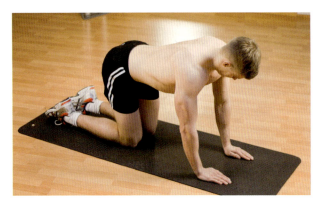 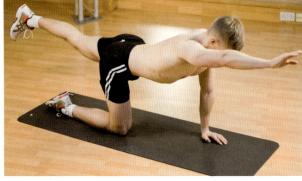

Starting Position:

Kneel on all fours, with knees under hips and hands under shoulders. Make sure you keep a small, inward curve in your low back. Keep your neck long, your shoulder blades down and your elbows unlocked.

Action:

Reach one arm forwards off the floor whilst simultaneously sliding the opposite foot along the floor away from the body. Continue to reach and raise the leg off the floor as far as control can be maintained through your pelvis and low back.

Repeat alternating arms and legs eight to 10 times.

Watch points
- Keep you neck long and deep abdominals activated throughout.
- Keep the correct curvature throughout the spine during the exercise.
- Lengthen and raise the leg by activating the buttocks.
- Imagine a glass of water on your back throughout the exercise.

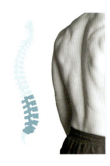

PLANK EXERCISE

Aim: To strengthen and stabilise the low back

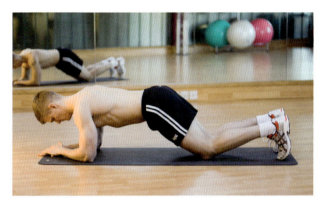 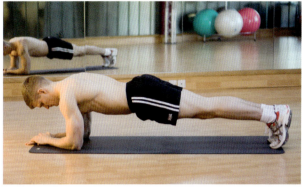

Starting Position:

Lie on your front propped up on your forearms, knees and toes.

Action:

Lift your pelvis and knees off the floor, creating a horizontal line from shoulders to ankles.
Hold for five to 10 seconds.

Repeat eight to 10 times.

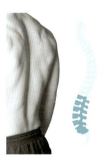

Watch points

- Do not allow your low back to dip down during the exercise.
- Keep your deep abdominals activated throughout.
- Use a mirror to check your alignment during the exercise.

Variations: If you find this difficult start by supporting your weight through the knees not the feet, over time gradually take your knees backwards

SIDE PLANK EXERCISE

Aim: To strengthen and stabilise the low back

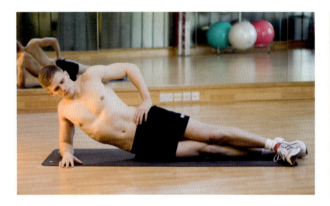 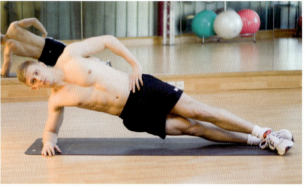

Starting Position:

Lie on your side supporting your upper body weight on your forearm and keeping a straight line from your shoulders to your ankles. Keep your neck long and shoulder blades down.

Action:

Raise your pelvis upwards until you achieve a straight line from shoulders to ankles. Hold for five to 10 seconds.

Repeat eight to 10 times.

Watch points
- Keep your pelvis forward throughout the exercise.
- Keep your deep abdominals activated throughout.
- Use a mirror to check your alignment during the exercise.

Variations: If you find this difficult start by supporting your weight through the knee not the feet.

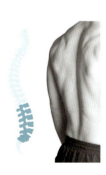

BUTTOCK & LEG STRETCHES

So far, your exercise programme has concentrated on strengthening and stretching your back and neck. But if you suffer from low back pain and leg pain, the tightness of your buttock and leg muscles may well be a contributing factor to your pain.

These exercises will help you to recognise tightness in specific muscles of the buttocks or legs and guide you in improving the flexibility of these muscles

It takes weeks or months to see the benefits of regular stretching, so patience and perseverance are important factors in your improvement regime.

Benefits of Buttock and Leg Stretches

✓ Improved flexibility of the leg muscles

✓ Less tension on the low back and sciatic nerve

✓ Improved posture

✓ Less discomfort in the legs and low back

✓ Greater ease in undertaking daily tasks

The Routine

■ Hold each stretch for 20-30 seconds whilst taking deep abdominal breathes

■ Repeat each stretch two to three times daily.

KNEELING QUAD STRETCH

Aim: To stretch the thigh and hip muscles

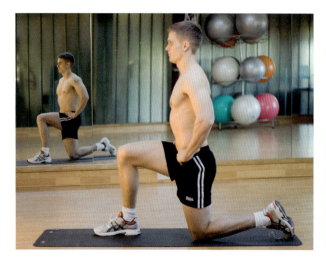 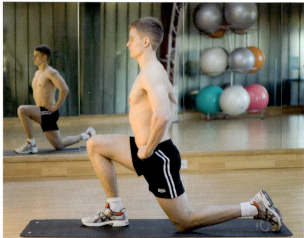

Technique

Kneel on one foot and the other knee. If needed, hold onto something to keep your balance. Keep your back straight and push your hips forward. Feel for a stretch in the front of the hip and thigh.
Hold for 20-30 seconds whilst taking deep breaths.

Repeat two to three times.

Watch points
- Place a pillow under your knee if needed for comfort.
- Keep your hips square throughout the exercise.
- Only stretch as far as is comfortable.

STANDING HAMSTRING STRETCH

Aim: To stretch and lengthen the hamstring muscles

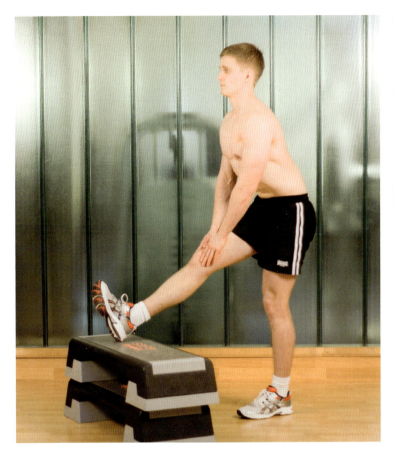

Technique

Stand upright and raise one leg on to an object. Keep that leg straight and your toes pointing straight up. Lean forward whilst keeping your back straight. Hold for 20-30 seconds whilst taking deep breaths.

Repeat two to three times.

Watch points
- ■ Only stretch as far as is comfortable.
- ■ Your low back should not arch at any time.

STANDING QUAD STRETCH

Aim: To stretch and lengthen the thigh muscles

Technique

Stand upright whilst balancing on one leg. Hold onto something for balance. Pull your other foot up behind your buttocks and keep your knees together whilst tucking your tailbone under and pushing your hips forward.
Hold for 20-30 seconds whilst taking deep breaths.

Repeat two to three times.

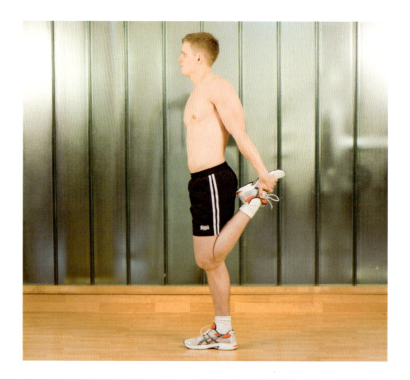

Watch points

- If you suffer from knee pain, avoid this stretch.
- Keep your knees together throughout the exercise.
- Do not lean forwards.
- Only stretch as far as is comfortable
- Hold onto the bottom of your trousers or hold onto a towel around your ankle to make the stretch easier

LEANING CALF STRETCH

Aim: To stretch and lengthen the calf muscles

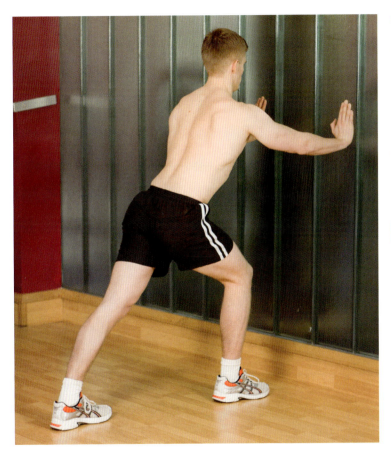

Technique

Stand upright and lean against a wall. Place one foot as far from the wall as is comfortable and make sure that both toes are facing forward and your heel is on the ground. Keep your back leg straight and lean forward.
Hold for 20-30 seconds whilst taking deep breaths.

Repeat two to three times.

Watch points
- Make sure the toes and foot of the back leg are facing forward.
- Only stretch as far as is comfortable.

LYING CROSS KNEE PULL UP STRETCH

Aim: To stretch and lengthen the buttocks

Technique

Lie on your back and cross on leg over the other. Bring your foot up to your opposite knee and with your opposite arm pull your raised knee up towards your chest.

Repeat two to three times.

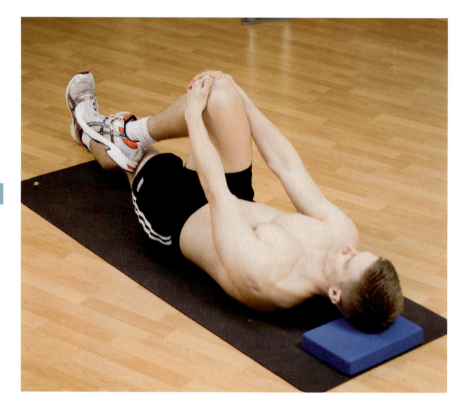

Watch points
- Keep both shoulders on the ground.
- Only stretch as far as is comfortable.

LYING DEEP GLUTEAL STRETCH

Aim: To stretch and lengthen the piriformis muscle

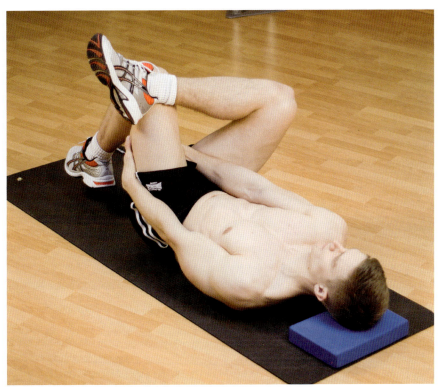

Technique

Lie on your back and bend one leg. Raise the other foot up onto the other leg and rest it on your thigh. Then reach forward holding onto your knee and pull towards you. Keep your tailbone on the floor throughout and your pelvis square. You should feel the stretch in the buttock of the leg resting on the other knee. This is a difficult stretch so use a towel around the knee if you are unable to perform the stretch

Hold for 20-30 seconds while taking deep breathes.

Repeat two to three times.

Watch points
- Only stretch as far as is comfortable.
- Do not let your tailbone tuck under you.
- Keep your pelvis square.

NECK EXERCISES

If you suffer from pain or muscular tension in the neck or shoulders then this is the section for you! You will learn how to identify your muscle tightness and how to stretch these areas. You will also learn strengthening exercises for the neck and shoulder blades to take the strain away from these painful areas.

Benefits of the Neck Exercises

✓ Improved posture

✓ Less discomfort in your neck and shoulders

✓ Less muscle tension around your shoulder blades

✓ Increased strength and endurance in your neck and shoulders

The Routine

■ Practise the stretches to identify your areas of muscle tightness, and do these exercises as recommended daily.

■ Work through the strengthening section and perform this routine every day.

■ Follow each exercise instruction and gradually increase to the recommended amount

■ Keep each motion slow and controlled

■ Remember to maintain abdominal breathing throughout the exercises.

TENSION RELIEVING NECK STRETCH

Aim: To reduce tension and stretch the neck

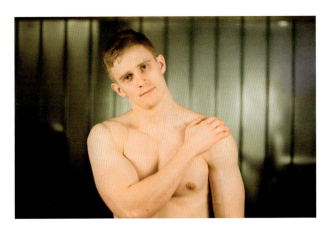

Starting Position:

Sit in a chair whilst keeping your shoulder blades down and your neck long. Place your left hand on your right shoulder.

Action:

Lower your left ear towards your left shoulder. Only stretch as far as is comfortable.
Hold for 20-30 seconds whilst taking deep abdominal breathes.

Repeat on alternating sides, 2 or 3 times each.

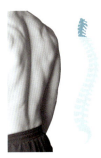

Watch points

- Use your hand to stop your shoulder from raising up during the exercise.
- Keep your neck long and shoulder blades down throughout.

Variations: Experiment during the stretch by rotating the head slightly to target tight areas within the muscle.
To help keep the shoulder down, hold underneath the chair or interlock the fingers behind the back.

FORWARD FLEXION NECK STRETCH

Aim: Forward Flexion Neck Stretch

Technique

Stand or sit upright. Now, slowly draw the chin inwards and then let your chin fall towards your chest. Keep your shoulder blades down and relaxed throughout. Hold for 20-30 seconds whilst taking deep breaths.

Repeat two to three times.

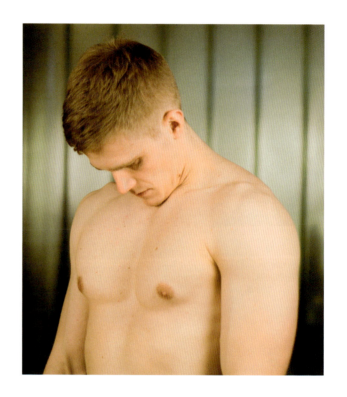

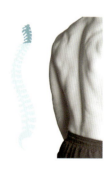

Watch points
- Do not overstretch by forcing your head down: let the weight of your head provide the necessary pressure
- Only stretch as far as is comfortable

NECK ROTATION STRETCH

Aim: To stretch the neck muscles and mobilise the joints in the neck and upper back

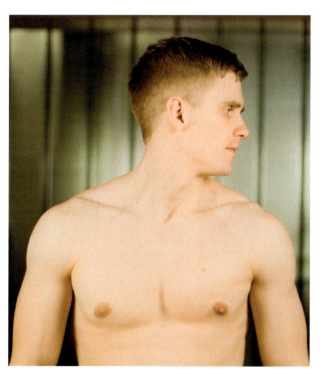

Technique

Stand or sit upright. Keep your shoulder blades down and relaxed. Slowly rotate your chin towards your opposite shoulder. Hold for 20-30 seconds whilst taking deep breaths.

Repeat two to three times.

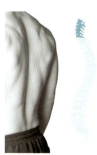

Watch points
- Keep your head up and do not let your chin fall towards your chest or shoulders
- Only stretch as far as is comfortable.

CHEST STRETCH

Aim: To improve posture and stretch the chest and upper shoulders

Starting Position:

Stand with your spine in correct alignment and your hands on your hips. Keep your neck long and shoulder blades down throughout the exercise.

Action:

Slowly pull your shoulders back and your elbows towards each other. Hold for 20-30 seconds. Slowly return to the starting position.

Repeat eight to 10 times.

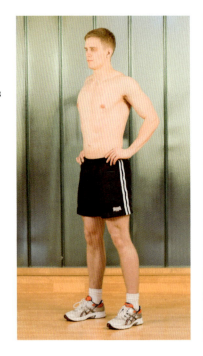
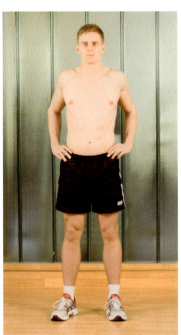

Watch points

- Do not arch your back during the exercise.
- Keep your neck long.
- Only stretch as far as is comfortable.

Variations: To progress the stretch, interlock your fingers behind your back, pull your shoulders back and lift your hands away from you.

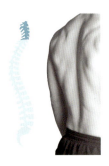

CHIN TUCKS

Aim: To reduce tension in the neck and strengthen the deep postural muscles

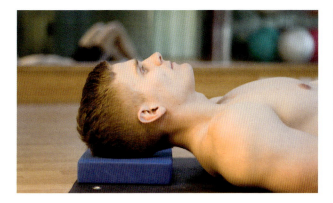

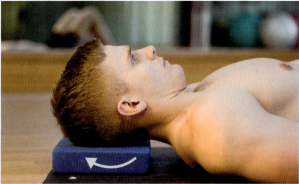

Starting Position:

Lie on your back on a mat or the carpet. Place a small, flat cushion or book under your head. Bend your knees and keep your feet straight and in line with your hips. Keep your chest and ribcage relaxed and your chin gently tucked in.

Action:

Gently lengthen the back of the neck feeling the chin slowly draw inwards. Hold for eight to 10 breaths.

Repeat up to 10 times.

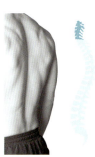

Watch points

- Make sure your head remains on the floor.
- Keep the large muscles on the front of the neck relaxed throughout.
- Ensure your movements are slow and smooth, not fast and jerky.
- Make sure your shoulders and chest remain relaxed.

Variations: After drawing the neck inwards, roll your neck slowly to the side. Never move into pain. Slowly return and repeat to the other side.

SHOULDER BLADE & NECK STRENGTHENING

Aim: To strengthen the postural muscles around the neck and shoulder blades and reduce muscle tension.

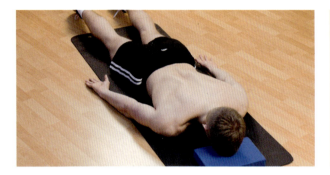
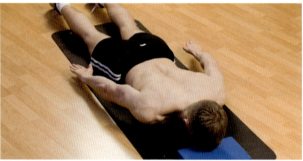

Starting Position:

Lie on your front with a small, folded towel or flat cushion under your forehead. Keep your neck long, as you do in the "Chin Tucks" exercise.

Action:

Slide your shoulder blades down into your back away from your ears. Hold for three to five breaths. Relax the shoulder blades to the starting position. The head remains down and the neck long.

Repeat eight to 10 times.

Watch points
- Do not squeeze your arms into your sides. Imagine you are holding a ripe peach between your arm and your body.
- Do not allow your low back to arch. Use a folded towel under your stomach to avoid this.
- Stop if you feel any pain in your neck or back.

Variations: To progress the exercise further, try hovering your hands one inch from the floor after sliding your shoulder blades down.
When you are comfortable with the previous variation, you can progress to simultaneously hovering the forehead one inch off the towel, keeping your neck long.

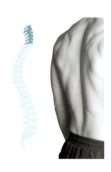

GENERAL AEROBIC EXERCISE PROGRAMME

This section is designed to start you off with a simple workout, consisting of straightforward aerobic exercises. This will build up your confidence and encourage you to return to the activities you enjoy. Increased activity will strengthen your back, help you sleep better at night, and have more energy during the day.

Benefits of the General Aerobic Exercise Programme

✓ Strengthens your entire body

✓ Lowers blood pressure

✓ Helps decrease stress

✓ Burn calories and speed up your metabolism

Slowly build up the time you spend doing aerobic exercise each week. Below are some exercise ideas, which you might enjoy.

- A brisk walk
- Cycling
- Swimming
- An elliptical machine in the gym
- An exercise class, such as Pilates or yoga

SQUAT

Aim: A great overall exercise to increase flexibility and strength to the spine and leg muscles

Starting Position:

Stand with your feet shoulder-width apart and feet facing forwards. Hold your hands straight out in front of you.

Action:

Bend your knees, and as you sink, sit back as if you were heading for a chair. Push your chest forward and keep your head up and looking straight in front of you. Do not let your knees push forward and aim to keep equal weight between the front and back of your feet. Go down as far as is comfortable, aiming so your thighs are parallel to the floor. Slowly rise back to the starting position.

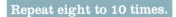

Repeat eight to 10 times.

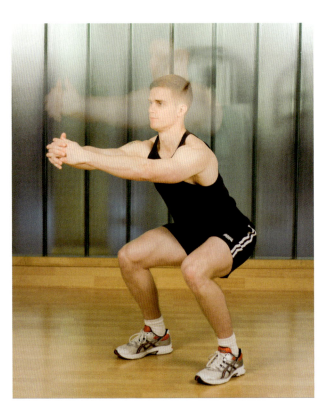

Watch points
- Always keep your heels on the floor and your spine in alignment.
- It may take weeks till your thighs are parallel to the floor, but make this one of your goals. This will increase your flexibility and strength to the spine and legs.
- Never bounce in the squat position.

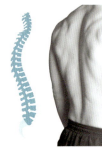

WALL PRESS UPS

Aim: To strengthen the upper body and spine

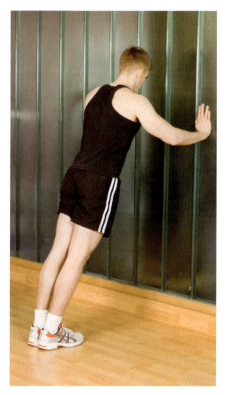

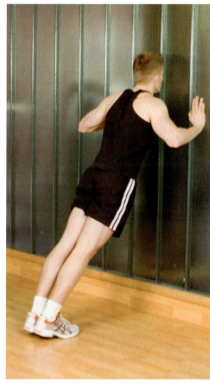

Starting Position:

Place your hands on a wall at shoulder height and just wider than shoulder-width apart. Your feet should be shoulder-width apart and positioned some distance away from the wall.

Action:

Keeping your chest and head up, take your chest down towards the wall, whilst keeping your legs in line with your spine. Slowly return to the starting position.

Repeat eight to 10 times.

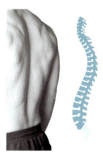

Watch points

- Keep your deep abdominals contracted throughout
- Do not bend from the waist
- To make the exercise harder, move your feet further away from the wall

STAR-SHAPED SIDE STEPS

Aim: A great aerobic exercise for the entire body

Starting Position:

Stand upright, with your arms at your sides.

Action:

Step sideways and in the same movement raise up the arms. Repeat five times on one side and then five times on the alternate side.

Repeat the sequence eight to 10 times on both sides.

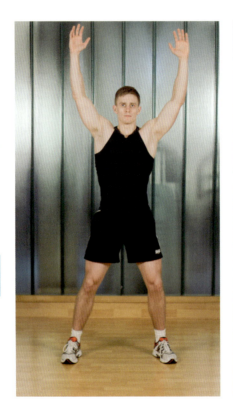
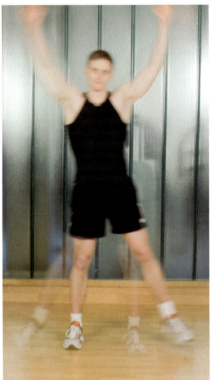

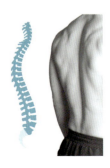

Watch points

- Keep your deep abdominals contracted throughout.
- If you have shoulder problems, use an alternate arm exercise.

HIGH KNEES

Aim: To improve balance and exercise the arms and legs

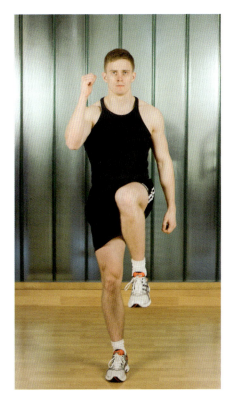 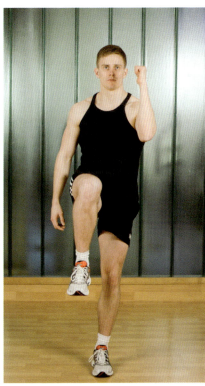

Starting Position:

Stand upright, with your arms at your sides.

Action:

Bring one knee up to the horizontal position whilst simultaneously bending the elbows into a bicep curl. Next, lower the leg and arms to the starting position, and then repeat for the other leg.

Repeat 10 –20 times with each leg.

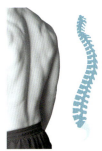

Watch points
- Keep your deep abdominals contracted throughout.
- Keep the pelvis and spine still throughout the exercise.
- Add hand weights to increase difficulty.

HEEL TO BOTTOM

Aim: To improve balance, spinal control and stretch the front of the legs.

Starting Position:

Stand upright, with your arms at your sides.

Action:

Bend one knee bringing the heel as far as possible up to the buttock, whilst simultaneously bending your elbows into a bicep curl. Return to the starting position and repeat for the other leg.

Repeat 10–20 times with each leg.

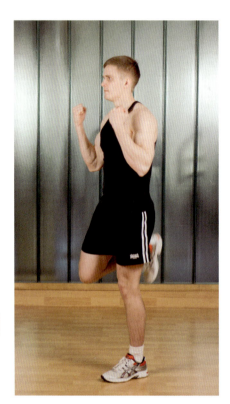
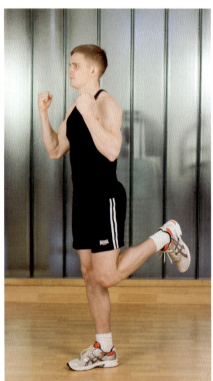

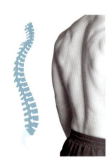

Watch points
- Keep your deep abdominals contracted throughout.
- Only stretch as far as is comfortable.
- Keep the pelvis and spine still throughout the exercise.

STEP UPS

Aim: To improve aerobic endurance and strengthen the back.

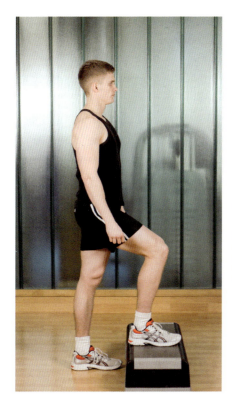 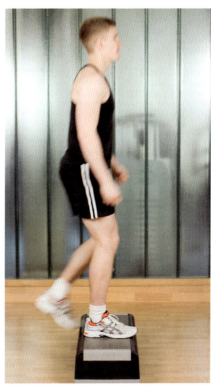

Starting Position:

Standing facing a step. If no step is available, use a few large books stacked against a wall.

Action:

Step up with one leg onto the step, followed by the other leg. Now step down using the leading leg, and then bring the other leg down to the starting position.

Step up and down 10-20 times leading with one leg, then change legs and repeat.

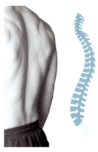

Watch points

- The slower you raise and lower the leg, the harder the muscles work.
- Keep the knee over the toes when stepping up.
- Keep your deep abdominals contracted throughout.
- Keep the pelvis and spine still throughout the exercise.

PARTING WORDS...

Modern medicine tells us that back pain is an inevitable part of growing older. It tells us that most of us will have to live with a degree of immobility and discomfort, and that all we can do is protect our backs by reducing our activity levels, taking extra care and living in fear of a recurrence.

This book has showed you that the conventional medical approach doesn't always work, and doesn't even make sense. Why would more and more of us be developing back problems in an age of better and better diagnostics, unless it was the diagnostics that were contributing to the problem? By creating fear, hopelessness and uncertainty, MRIs, X-rays and other diagnostic tools are actually contributing to the epidemic. Many of us are caught in a cycle of fear, stress-related pain and recurrence.

But now you have the tools and knowledge you need to end that cycle and improve your health—now and forever. Your secret weapon is your mental approach. When you understand that you have the power to control your pain, everything changes. By recognising and understanding the impact repressed emotions such as fear, anger and frustration can have on your health, you can realign the mind-body connection and dissolve emotionally triggered pain. You don't have to feel vulnerable and helpless about your back pain any more. In fact, it's integral to your recovery that you conquer those feelings!

You have the power to change your physical health. This book has placed that power in your hands. Now all you need to do is follow the steps, commit to the exercise programme, and work to keep a positive mindset.

I wish you all the best in your journey to complete recovery from pain!

Nick Sinfield has many years of experience in treating back and neck pain patients within the United Kingdom and New Zealand. He has worked within the public and private sectors, which has helped to broaden his knowledge and practical experience.

As well as being a registered physiotherapist, he is a qualified Pilates instructor with certification from the Australian Physiotherapy Pilates Institute. This interdisciplinary approach to physical health has given him a unique perspective and valuable complementary knowledge in the area of back and neck strengthening.

He currently spends his working time treating patients at clinics in Bedfordshire, Hertfordshire and in high-level rugby.

Nick Sinfield is registered with the Health Professions Council and a member of the Chartered Society of Physiotherapy.

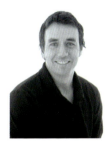

Nick Sinfield MCSP, HPC, APPI

SHORT-TERM GOALS

LONG-TERM GOALS

....
....
....
....
....
....
....
....
....
....
....
....
....
....
....
....
....
....
....
....
....

NOTES